ZERO MINUTE YOGA

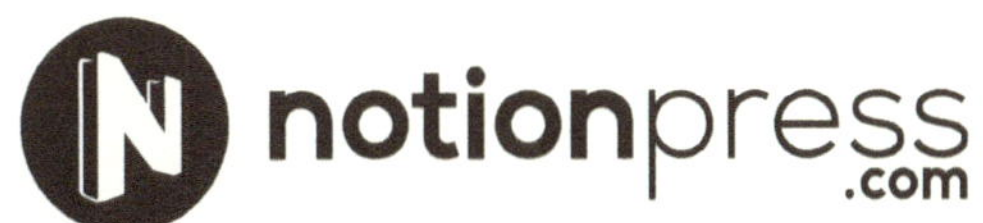

ZERO MINUTE YOGA
CUTTING THE ROOTS OF DISEASES

BIDHYA BHUSAN SINGH

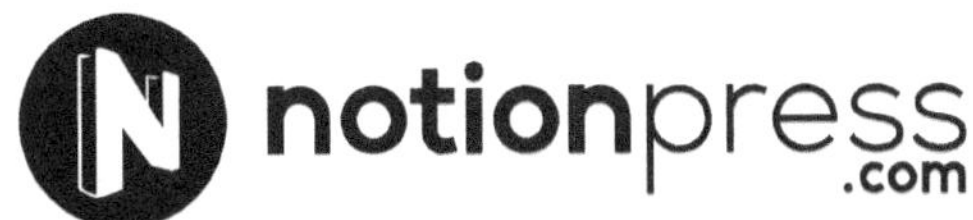

Notion Press

Old No. 38, New No. 6
McNichols Road, Chetpet
Chennai - 600 031

First Published by Notion Press 2016
Copyright © Bidhya Bhusan Singh 2016
All Rights Reserved.

ISBN 978-1-946048-90-5

Contents

Preface

Zero Minute Yoga is for those who are busy, and cannot spare time to practice yoga, but still wish to remain healthy and cure their ailments through yoga. A lot of research validated the importance of yoga in the field of health and diseases. Some unsolved questions like wave-particle duality, phenomenon of entanglement etc., have forced scientists to accept the philosophical dimensions of yoga. Further, the concept of noosphere (the sphere of human thought), Rupert Sheldrake's morphic resonance (collective memory), Vedic Akashic library and Carl Jung's collective unconscious, reflect the unity of the universe and its interacting features.

To benefit from yoga, it must be understood in its entirety. Some emphasise on physical postures and others on the mental aspects or meditation. Yoga is a practice and merely knowing its higher philosophy does not give much benefit. Body is the centre through which anything can be perceived, enjoyed and achieved. So Yoga gives importance to maintain a healthy body and mind. Body and mind are not two different things. Each cell in our body is an independent identity. Individual cells have very elaborate communication system and human cells use thousands of signals to communicate with each other. Recently, it has been found that cells are able to communicate with photons from cell to cell. In the 1990s, according to Dr Horowitz, "three Nobel laureates in medicine did advance research that revealed the primary function of DNA lies not in protein synthesis… but in the realm of bioacoustic and bioelectric signaling."

"From a Cymatics or vibratory standpoint, disharmony is disease. The critical concept to grasp here is that all manifestations of disease, whether diagnosed as "physiological" or "psychological," result from disruption (in the form of toxicity or trauma) of the primary electromagnetic harmonies and rhythm contained in the auric fields and corresponding chakras. These bioenergy centers have an intimate relationship with DNA that gives them direct regulatory access to all cellular functions. Therefore, if we can find a way to reset our bioenergy blueprint through harmonic resonance, we can go directly to the root of disease processes." – Sol Luckman. The purpose of yoga is to synchronise the whole body and to remove blockages of energy so that each cell can communicate and remain in harmony.

Human civilization has moved from a hunter-gatherer lifestyle to a sedentary lifestyle, which has resulted in many health problems and diseases. Modern way of life is less physically active and a wide range of labour-saving devices reduced the physical demand. Unnatural diets, pollution and stress increased the susceptibility to many diseases. Asanas or yogic body postures give the benefit of relaxation, stretching and strengthening at the same time.

When I started teaching yoga through yoga camps and in classes, I emphasised on meditative aspects of yoga and I found that people were in hurry to cure their various ailments. Many people used to come with their diseases, and ask about asanas that could possibly cure them. Keeping these facts in mind, a short form of yogic practices is scheduled in such a way that it can be included in the daily routine and does not take extra time or a yoga mat for practice. Though short in form, *Zero Minute Yoga* (ZMY) includes all aspects of yoga from purification to meditation, and helps in eliminating many diseases. I initially brought it in the form of a pamphlet and distributed it, which gave me very positive feedback. Suggestions came in to bring it in the form of a book, which I have now managed to do. ZMY cured many people, freed them from diseases and it will prove to be a boon and will revolutionise the health system.

This book has three Sections: Basics, Zero Minute Yoga and Beyond Zero Minute Yoga. In Basics, the theory behind Zero Minute Yoga has been explained. The section on Zero Minute Yoga provides details on yogic practices and how to include it in our daily routine. Finally, in Beyond Zero Minute Yoga, some higher aspects of yogic concepts have been explained to prepare the reader for understanding the subtle nuances of yoga.

BASICS

ZMY

(Introduction)

Zero Minute Yoga attempts to encourage including yogic kriyas in our daily routine, so that extra time or space are not required. Instructions on how to perform ZMY have been given in the chapter 'How to do Zero Minute Yoga', so read it carefully before starting your yogic practice.

Hatha yoga gives much importance to the purification of the body. Purification processes or Satkarma (six processes) prepare the body for further yogic kriyas such as asanas, pranayam, meditation etc. In Zero Minute Yoga, one important method of body cleansing, Sankha Prakshalan, has been shortened and explained for daily use, to keep the body free from accumulation of toxins.

In Ayurvedic and Naturopathy system of therapy, more emphasis has been given to abdominal cleansing. According to the traditional Chinese belief, the Gut is the 'foundation for human health.' The abdomen is the centre, where toxins accumulate due to undigested food caused by modern-day diets and different types of stress. Constipation is not the only a bowel problem, but the root of all diseases like skin-related problems including eczema, psoriasis, acne, and lung-related issues like asthma, bronchitis, sinusitis, and brain related like memory loss and many others.

In Kundalini yoga, the abdomen is the place of the manipur chakra or solar plexus. Manipur chakra is the master of the physical body and keeps its symbol fire or digestive fire burning. Zero Minute Yoga targets the abdomen to keep the body healthy and frees it from different types of diseases.

All aspects of yoga are included in this Zero Minute Yoga. T. T. K is a part of Shatkarma or Purification. The Boat and Reverse Boat Pose are very important and are curative asanas. Anulom Vilom Pranayam is the most important and beneficial pranayam and meditation given in Zero Minute format is easy for beginners and it prepares for higher level of meditation.

Yoga and Therapy

Diseases have become synonymous with day to day life. Even before birth, a baby has to go through so many medications. Scientific progress has given many things to the modern civilization, and people come to know the mysteries of universal laws and it has contributed a lot in the health sector, but a number of diseases were on the rise and were named as lifestyle diseases. Here, emerged the need of an alternative way to save the diseased world and people began to move towards ancient wisdom for the solution.

Though Yoga is not a pure science of therapy, mental and physical fitness are the crux of yoga. In yoga, we are part of the whole universe and the purpose of life is to connect with the universe again. For this connection, we have to come out of our worldly connection.

To become complete, or whole, you have to finish the very existence of 'me', only then a drop of water after losing its existence becomes the ocean. To reach the higher goal of yoga or becoming one with the universe you have to prepare your body and mind.

To prepare ourselves for the higher side of yoga, we have to pass through the purification process of our body. This purification process of yoga has been taken and utilized for therapeutic use. There are many types of yogic methods and the important ones among them are Hatha yoga and Raja yoga. In Hatha yoga, there is Shatkarma kriya or six processes of body purification to prepare for yoga kriyas (process). In Raja yoga, there are eight limbs that is stage by stage to reach the higher stage of self-realization. Diseases are the manifestation of imbalance and first occur at the subtle body or pranic body.

In Hatha yoga, the importance of Satkarma is to purify the body and free it from diseases. They are Neti, Dhauti, Nauli, Basti, Tratak, and Kapalbhati. Through these Kriyas, different parts of the body and emotions are purified.

Yama, Niyama, Asana, Pranayam, Pratyahara, Dharana, Dhyan, and Samadhi are the eight stages of Raja yoga. Through the first four stages, the body and mind are purified and prepared for the higher side of yoga in the next four stages.

Modern science tried to study these aspects of yoga, and found it to be beneficial for the well-being of human beings. The body is a playground of hormones, chemicals, neurons, and their activities are affected by many external factors such as emotions, exercise, environment etc.

In these complex interactions, yoga is regarded as a safe method to remain healthy, physically and mentally. Yoga is not only preventive but curative, as proved by modern research. That is the reason why yoga has become popular as a treatment for the growing number of diseases in the world. According to Bruce Lipton – "Most illness is just from the stress of not living in harmony." Again he says that at theta level (Theta brain waves), changes occur in the DNA, which can affect any aspect of one's physical health. Stress is not a minor problem; it has an immense influence on our genetic expression. It is not only an everyday stress, but our body and mind carry the cellular memory of the stress of our ancestors, and the tensions of the mother and child, while in the mother's womb. It is through meditation and continuous relaxation that those memories of the past are erased slowly, and we come out of those stresses and progress towards regeneration of the body and mind on a cellular level.

Complexity biology contains words such as fractural Physiology, criticality and self-organized criticality. When the mind is deprived of information, body gets rest and it puts itself back into a state of health. Physical laws can always be trumped by non-physical powers. In every physical system, the law of entropy dictates that energy will dissipate over time, but life is the prime example of negative entropy which counters the law of entropy. The play of entropy (disintegration) and centropy (integration) continues throughout life. Yoga prepares and protects the body from the laws of entropy.

The feedback I received from my yoga camps and classes confirmed the therapeutic dimension of yoga. In camps and classes, I teach more asanas and pranayamas but Zero Minute Yoga remains in the centre. Most of the practitioners became disease free. Experiences of some of the practitioners are given below:

- A major accident almost paralysed me with many broken bones. I came out of a long period of coma with the help of medical intervention, but I was not in a position to walk independently. The wheelchair became a part of my life. Sir taught me some yoga which I did regularly, and slowly I became independent. Now I have no need of support or wheelchairs and can move freely and do my job.

  Md. Shamim

- I am eighty-two years old. I was suffering from hypertension, asthma and other age related problems and weakness. After doing yoga, all my problems are solved and now I feel like a sixteen-year-old boy. Medicines are stopped which saved my money also.

  Baleswar Prasad Singh

- I attended the yoga camp and did it regularly under the guidance of Sri Bidhya Bhusan Singh whom we call Sir or Guruji (Spiritual guide). I was suffering from hypertension, hypothyroidism and diabetes. Now I am completely free from diseases and medicines and now there is no need to consult a doctor. I suggest everyone to do yoga.

  Ved Prakash Agarwal

- My body was stiff; legs were almost paralysed and I was unable to walk smoothly. I joined the yoga camp and started doing it regularly under the guidance of Sir. Now I am completely cured. From a burden on my family, I have become capable of carrying the burden of my family.

  Ranjit Kumar Gupta

- After joining Yoga Camp I feel that yoga is an integral part of life. It eliminated my weakness, laziness and irritation and cured my hypothyroidism problem. It proved a boon for me and changed my life.

  Bhikhari Ram

- I am a seventy-two-year-old lady. I was suffering from tiredness, breathlessness, joint pain, insomnia, hypothyroidism, low blood pressure and many other problems. After joining Yoga Camp under Guruji (Bidhya Bhusan Singh), all my problems vanished and now I am fully cured and feel like a young lady.

  Heera Muni Devi

- I was suffering from many types of ailments such as obesity, hypothyroidism, recurring E. coli, irritable bowel syndrome and other related problems. Yoga, under guidance of Sri Bidhya Bhusan Singh made me physically active and disease free. I advise him to expand his activity so that more and more people can benefit from Yoga

  Dr Anita Rani Singh

These are a few examples. Many people did only TTK, some did only Boat Pose and they got the benefits of yoga. Dedication and continuous practice gives results.

Gut

The Central focus of Zero Minute Yoga is on gastrointestinal tract, also known as the Gut or alimentary canal. That is why it becomes necessary to know in brief the importance of Gut in maintaining physical and mental health. Gut is also called the second brain because it contains nearly a 100 million neurons, and almost independently does its work of digestion. The Gut produces 95% of the body's serotonin, the happy hormone in our body, and so an unhealthy Gut affects mood. 70-80% of immune system is located in the digestive system and protects us from inflammatory diseases, cause behind almost all diseases.

Our bodies compromise about 100 trillion microbes in different parts of the body especially our Guts. These microbes or microbiota, play important role in regulating our immune systems, food digestion, manufacturing Vitamins and affecting everything from our mental health to our weight and changes to the Gut microbiome can precipitate disease. These changes occur due to wrong types of food and explosive use of antibiotics.

To restore Gut microbiota for curing many types of physical and mental illness, transplanting the stool from one person into the digestive tract of another person called Fecal Microbiota transplant or FMT is becoming popular and effective. The majority of the matter in stool, around 60% is bacteria. In China, during the sixteenth century, stool known as yellow soup was used for digestive problems. A German physician, Christian Franz Paullini, used stool for treating dysentery and other digestive problems during the seventeenth century.

The study shows that the more diverse your diet is, the more diverse the microbiome will be, and it will also be more immune to foreign particles. Dr Rupali Datta, Clinical Dietician at Fortis-Escorts Hospital suggests some healthy habits to strengthen your gut, "To start with, eat more fiber, it acts as a probiotic for the gut. Eat in a relaxed atmosphere, chew slowly, relish your food and have regular meal timings. These simple habits can really make a difference. You just need to make them a part of your daily routine. Make breakfast, your heaviest meal of the day and eat dinner before eight for smooth digestive functions"

Gut bacteria has a very important role to play in obesity, and unrestricted use of antibiotics is linked to the rising tide of human obesity. Since the 1940s farmers have been feeding their livestock antibiotics to promote rapid weight gain.

The Gut has its own brain, known as the enteric nervous system, plays a major role in human health. The Gut's brain is located in sheaths of tissue linking the esophagus, stomach, small intestine and colon. It is a complex circuitry like proper brain and has a network of neurons, neurotransmitters and proteins that enables it to act independently, learn and remember.

"Nearly every substance that helps run and control the brain has turned up in the Gut," Dr Michael Gershon said. Major neurotransmitters like serotonin, norepinephrine, nitric oxide, glutamate and dopamine exist there. Many brain proteins, called neuropeptides, are in the Gut. Major cells of the immune system are located in the Gut. Body's natural opiates and psychoactive chemicals are in the Gut.

Central nervous system and enteric nervous system are connected via a cable called the vagus nerve. The Gut contains 100 million neurons more than the spinal cord has.

Gut-Brain is like two-way traffic. The Gut can upset the brain just as the brain can upset the Gut. Patients with bowel problems have been shown to have abnormal REM sleep and known with folk wisdom that indigestion can produce nightmares. Patients of Alzheimer's and Parkinson's diseases suffer from constipation. Many autoimmune diseases like Krohn's disease and ulcerative colitis involve the gut's brain.

A new field of study called neurogastroenterology, emerged to know the interactions of the brain and gut and its role in different types of diseases.

These are the reasons why ancient therapeutic system emphasised so much on Gut health.

Backward Bending

Most people experience back pain at some point in their lives. Sedentary habits and desk job work create tension in the back, long hours of standing and athletic activities also create tension in the back. Hamstring muscles and iliopsoas get shortened which cause strain on the lower back.

The spinal column is a 'stacked pile' of vertebrae and discs. To keep the spine in a straight and aligned position depends on the balanced, supportive contraction and tone of the muscles which are controlled unconsciously through posture.

Swadhisthan Chakra is situated in the lower part of the vertebrae which is the centre of emotion. Subconscious tensions are reflected in the activity of the back muscles.

Tension in the back muscles create muscular imbalance resulting in backache and misalignment of vertebral column. Many diseases like osteoarthritis, spondylitis, slipped disc and sciatica are its manifestation.

The backward bending asanas, stretch the back and abdominal muscles which tone and strengthen the muscles controlling the spine. These nerves give energy to all other nerves, organs and muscles in the body and help in maintaining a healthy body. These asanas massage the abdomen and pelvic organs by stretching the muscles in these areas and correct the postural defects and neuromuscular imbalances of the vertebral column. Reverse Boat pose given in ZMY helps in correcting the posture and curing the problems of the back.

Pranayam

Pranayam is more than a simple breathing exercise. Prana is the vital life force and Pranayam is comprised of two words prana (life force) and ayama (expansion or lengthening), which means to expand the pranic force. Breathing is a direct means of absorbing prana and by manipulating it pranic vibrations are synchronized to influence our being. Prana and mind are interlinked, and when either the mind or prana becomes balanced, the other is steadied. The entire nervous system gets strengthened by the practice of Pranayam, which in turn leads to the soundness of the body and mind. According to an ancient scripture "Just as the impurities of metals (gold etc.) are removed by the flame of fire, the Indriyas (organs) throw out their impurities through Pranayam." Sage Patanjali says that Pranayam removes the obstacles of yoga.

In Pranayam, inhalation is called Purak, exhalation is called Rechak and the pause between inhalation and exhalation is called Kumbhak. Pause or retention of breath known as Kumbhak is a very powerful practice and is generally avoided.

There are many types of Pranayam but in ZMY, the most effective and simple Pranayam for curing diseases called Anulom-Vilom or Nadishodhan, has been given. Again Anulom-vilom has many variations. After perfecting this variation of ZMY, advance variations with breath retention can be done.

Meditation

Meditation has become a therapeutic word, as it has many positive effects on health, as proved by modern research. Pure scientific studies show that meditation changes our bodies on a genetic level. Stress is the major cause of diseases, as proved by modern studies. Stress disturbs the rhythm of the body and mind by keeping it in fight or flight mode. The whole physical system remains in hormonal imbalance, and hardly finds any time to balance it, which results in many types of diseases. In this restless world, meditation balances our emotions and gives deep relaxation, which brings back the body and mind in rhythm and works as a universal medicine to cure the imbalances of our body and frees it from different types of diseases.

Besides, altering the functions of our brain and body meditation also purifies our consciousness which influences the physical material world. Recent research clearly demonstrates that consciousness and the material physical world are directly intertwined. Quantum entanglement, collapse of the wave function etc., forced the new physics to admit that the observer creates the reality. The sciences of prayer, distance healing, blessings etc., have become the modern areas of study for the physicists, neuroscientists and psychologists.

Meditation regrows grey matter, the part of the brain that helps keep memory working. Meditation improves the very wiring of our brains by growing new, stronger neural connections.

Yoga is actually meditation and science of the mind. Ancient scriptures on yoga defined it as restraining the fluctuations of the mind. In Rig Veda, one who donates (calms) the mind is the performer of Yoga. Bhagavad Gita and Yoga Vasistha also defined yoga as, to remain in a neutral state without any fluctuation of the mind. Patanjali in Yoga sutra defined it as, Yoga is to restraint the tendencies of the mind. Chapter III, Sutra 39 of Siva Sutra says that as in the case of the states of the mind, so also in the case of the body, organs of sense, and external things, there should be vitalization with the bliss of the transcendental consciousness. The same has been said in *Vijnanabhairava:* "One should consider the whole world or one's own body, as filled with the bliss of the self. All at once with the nectar of one's own consciousness, he would be filled with the highest bliss." – Verse 65. Charaka, an ancient Indian physician, considers grief (Visada) as the potent cause of aggravator of diseases, cheerfulness (Harsa) as the best nourishing agent and worry (Soka) as the most important cause for extreme weakness.

The importance of discipline of the mind is in the centre of Yoga without which we cannot taste the nectar of Yoga and will remain on the periphery of it.

Now the question arises as to how to meditate. There are many ways shown by ancient and some modern thinkers to do meditation. Here in ZMY, a very simple method is given to discipline the mind to develop a passive attitude and prepare it for higher level of meditation. Therapeutically, this simple method is very effective in giving positive results.

Diseases-its Roots

To remain healthy, it is necessary to understand the root causes of diseases. Diseases are the manifestation of imbalance created in the body. Diseases are branches of a tree which cannot be eliminated by cutting the branches. Eastern systems like Ayurveda and Yoga, attack the root of a tree and branches fall down automatically.

In Ayurveda, Aama or undigested food is the major cause of disease. This Aama enters the system and creates disturbances in the proper functioning of different systems of the body. This causes accumulation of toxins in the body. The formation of Aama is due to the impaired state of Agni (Digestive fire). An analogy may be given to understand the relation between Aama and Agni. If rice is boiled at an optimum temperature for an optimum time, rice gets cooked. If the heat is insufficient or inconsistent (Sometimes too fierce, sometime too dull), then rice in the vessel does not get completely cooked. Like rice, food in the abdomen does not digest completely due to disturbed Agni (Digestive fire). Fasting allows the digestive system to rest. During fasting, the digestive fire rekindles, and this fire slowly burns away long-existing ama or toxins in the intestines. Fasting is usually adviced in fever, constipation, cold and arthritis. A warm water fast is advisable at least once a week for a normal healthy individual. According to Benjamin Franklin, "The best of all medicines are rest and fasting."

Stress is the other major cause of diseases. In stress, body pumps adrenaline, and then cortisol into the bloodstream to prepare the body and mind for immediate action. But when chronic stress exposes the body to a relentless stream of cortisol, it begins to create many problems in the body. Though cortisol turns off inflammation, its continuous flow desensitizes the cells "causing inflammation to go wild" as Cohen says. Long-term chronic inflammation causes many diseases in the body. According to Sri Sri Paramahansa Yogananda, "Stubborn mental or physical diseases always have a deep root in the subconsciousness. Illness may be cured by pulling out its hidden roots. That is why all affirmations of the conscious mind should be impressive enough to permeate the subconsciousness, which in turn automatically influences the conscious mind. Strong conscious affirmations thus react on the mind and body through the medium of the subconscious. Still stronger affirmations reach not only the subconscious, but also the superconscious mind – the magic storehouse of miraculous powers."

To discipline the mind or cortical monkey is very difficult. Abhyasa vairagyabhyam tannirodhah (Patanjali yogasutra 1/12) Practice and detachment restrain it. Lahiri mahasya used to say, "Banat, banat, ban jaye – doing, doing, at last, done." Regular attempts to restrain the fluctuations of the mind help in stilling the mind. Another very important word in Indian philosophy is vairagya (non-attachment or dispassion or indifference to sensual objects). Attachment creates Raga and Dvesha (likes and dislikes). Too much attachment to an object disturbs the thought-wave. Raga-Dvesha is the real cause of all diseases. In this world of stress and speed the understanding of these things thin out the attachment to a great extent.

ZMY balances Agni (Digestive fire), eliminates toxins and releases tension. Eat according to your digestive power, and try to minimize stress from your life. Perform yoga in a relaxed and meditative mode to get maximum benefit. Iccha Saktir Uma Kumari (Siva Sutra I/13) The willpower is the virgin light. Thought is like a seed. Always remain careful in choosing your thought or seed.

ZERO MINUTE YOGA

ZMY with Some Suggestions.

1. Body is the centre and only through a healthy body you can enjoy your life.
2. Keep children aware about their health. Yoga prepares them to fight against many diseases and stress.
3. Keep control over your eating habits. Chew your food completely and eat slowly, drink water after an hour. Eat your food two hours before going to bed.
4. Try to remain in a happy mood, create compassion and loving thoughts within yourself.

    It balances your immune system.
5. Restrict the use of salt, sugar, onion and garlic. They increase anxiety and are provocative in nature.

In recent times, people have not been paying much attention to their health due to too much engagement. Keeping these facts in view, this Zero Minute Yoga is presented in a very short form. The whole world is getting the benefit of yoga. Through Zero Minute Yoga, you can keep your body healthy and energetic and can protect yourself from diseases and doctors. It is beneficial for modern-day diseases like hypertension and diabetes.

Asana vs Exercise

Before starting Zero Minute Yoga, understanding the nuances of Asana is necessary. Asanas have often been thought of as a form of exercise. Exercise involves the body while Asana involves both the body and the mind. Asanas are done after calming the mind in a relaxed way and often with closed eyes. Body and mind are not separate entities. Body is the gross form of the mind while the mind is the subtle form of the body. The practice of Asanas synchronises and harmonises the body and the mind.

Asana in Sanskrit means a 'chair' or a 'seat', and in terms of bodily postures implies a seated pose. Patanjali says "Sthiram Sukham aasanam," meaning, 'to remain steady in a comfortable position'. Meditation, in classical yoga, requires the ability to sit comfortably for an extended period of time. In broader terms, Asanas developed into the forms of different body postures.

Asanas open the energy channels and psychic centres of the body and mind. Tension or mental knots create stiffness in the body which blocks the flow of prana or vital energy and a subsequent accumulation of toxins in the body. Asanas release this tension, remove toxins from the body and open the energy channels of the body. Regular practice of asana promotes health, releases day to day stress and makes our bodies disease free. It releases dormant energy and increases confidence in all areas of life. Hatha yoga Pradipika says 'Prior to everything, asana is spoken of as the first part of hatha yoga. Having done asana, one attains steadiness of body and mind, freedom from disease and lightness of the limbs.'

When Asanas are done in a relaxed and meditative mode its benefits increase many times. Yoga postures tend to arrest catabolism whereas exercise promotes it. Asanas make the body supple while exercises stiffen the body. Through asana, body gets the benefit of relaxation, stretching and strengthening at the same time.

How to do Zero Minute Yoga

Check the capacity and power of your body before starting yoga and move gradually according to the capacity of your body.

- First, after waking up in the morning, do the Boat Pose five times and Reverse Boat Pose two times on your bed.
- Before defecating, drink 1 L or more water according to your capacity, then do Tadasan, Triyak Tadasan and Kati chakrasan ten times each or less if weak, then defecate; it will wash your alimentary canal properly.
- Sit somewhere comfortably and do Anulom-Vilom five rounds. Meditate after it.
- These activities do not take extra time and keep you healthy mentally and physically.

Naukasana
(Boat Pose)

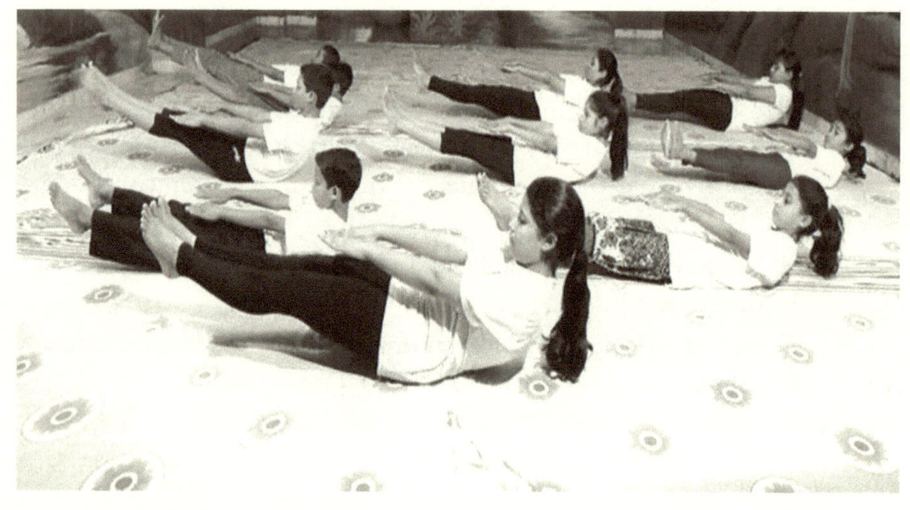

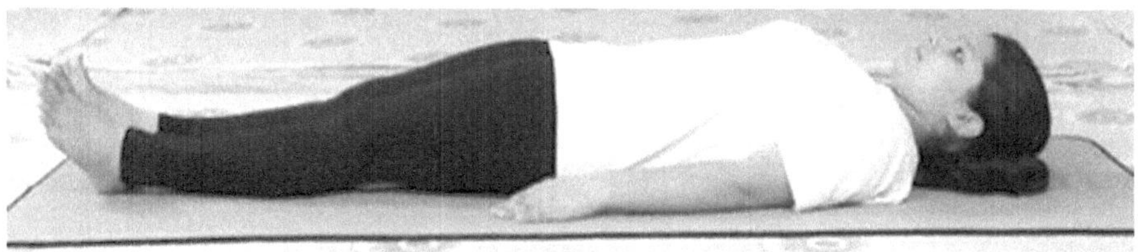

Step I

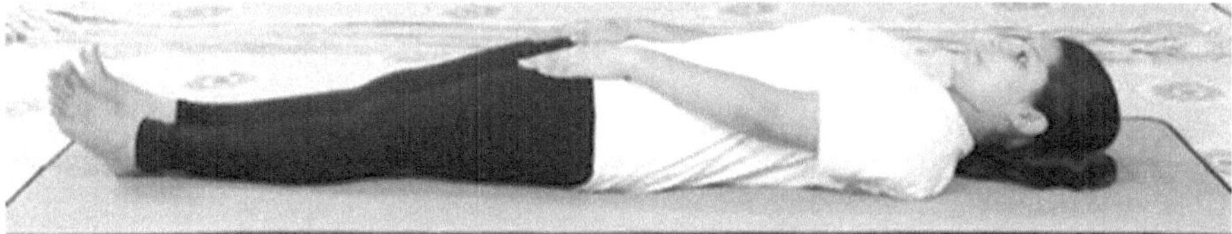

Step II

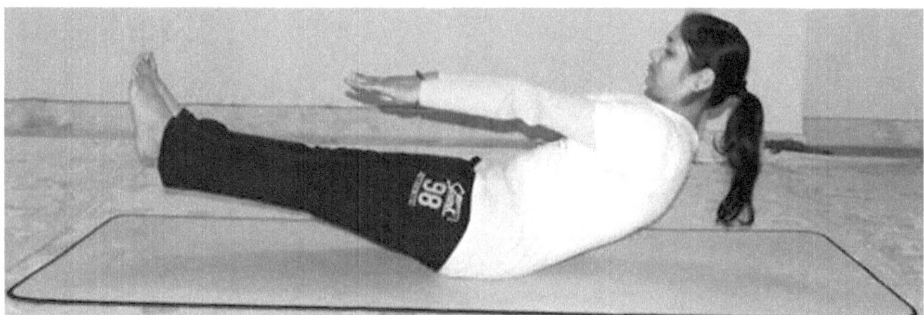

Final

Lie on the back keeping your arms on the thighs with your palms facing downwards. While inhaling, raise your legs, trunk, arms, and head about 15 cm and try to balance on the buttocks. Keep arms at the same level and in line with the toes. Remain in this position as long as retention of breath is comfortable. Slowly exhale, lower the body and relax. Do it five times.

Navel is the centre of the body. It is necessary to keep it in the centre for good health. Abdomen has its own brain which is called the second brain. Abdomen is also the source of the hormone serotonin, which keeps you happy. Gut bacteria has a very important role to play on your body and mind. Boat pose has a good effect on your liver, kidney, pancreas, spleen, prostrate, urinary bladder etc.

It has a curative effect on intestinal worms and good for the stutters. It relaxes the whole body and ultimately, the mind. Try to make this asana your daily habit, it can eliminate many internal problems.

Viprit Naukasana
(Reverse Boat Pose)

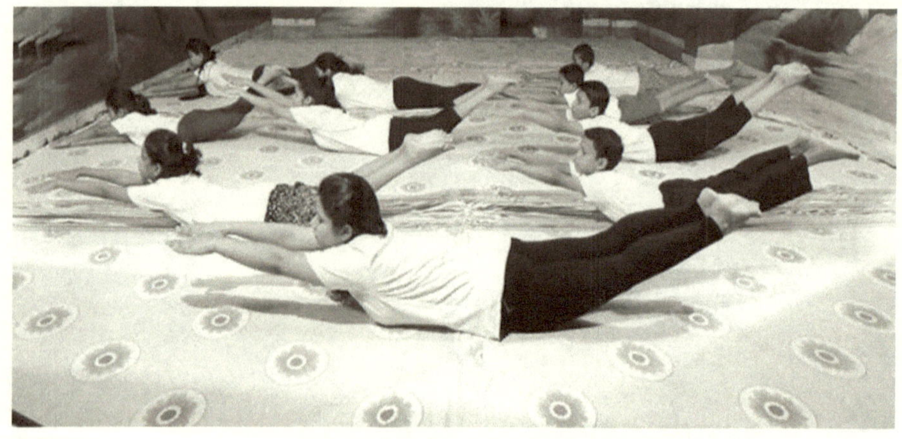

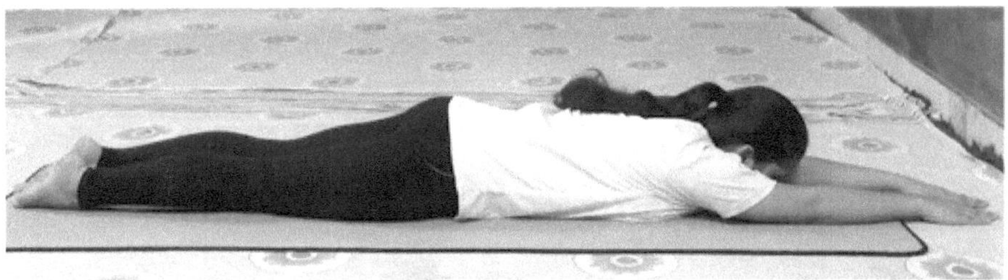

Step I

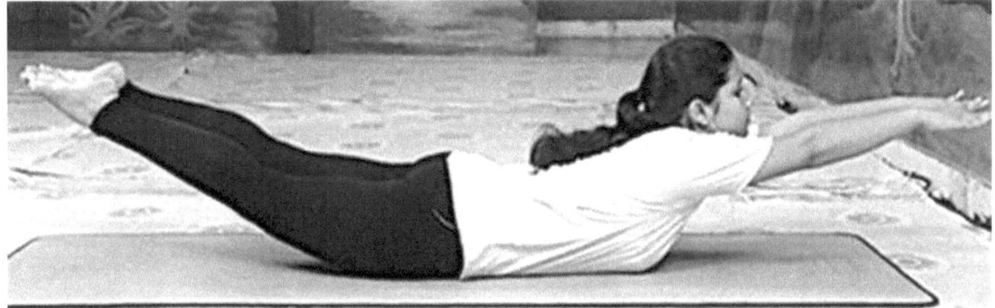

Final

Lie on your abdomen. Keep both your hands in front of your shoulder. Now raise your both hands and both legs so that the weight of whole body comes on your navel. Hold it for 10 seconds and then return to the original position. It has a curative effect on the neck, back and the waist pain.

Tadasan (Palm Tree Pose)

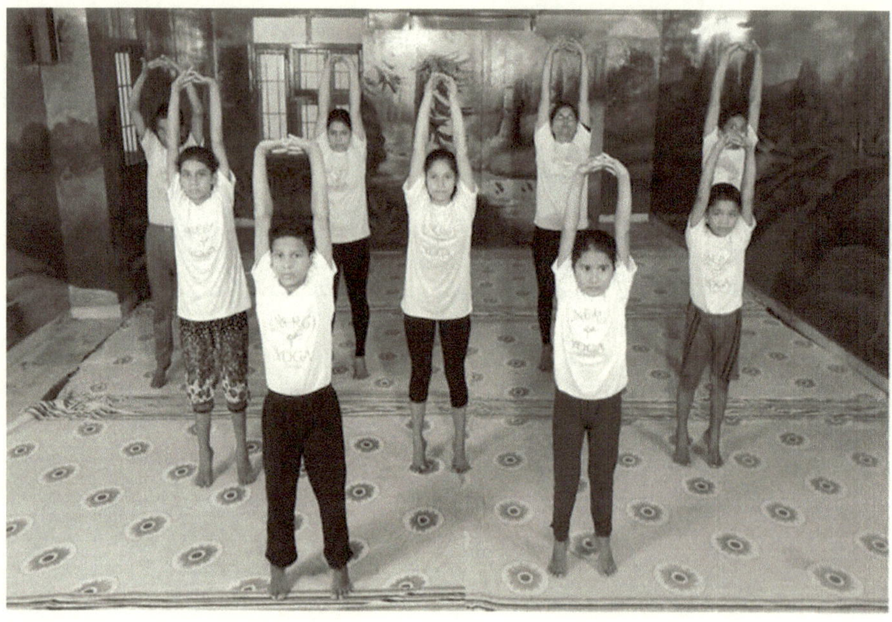

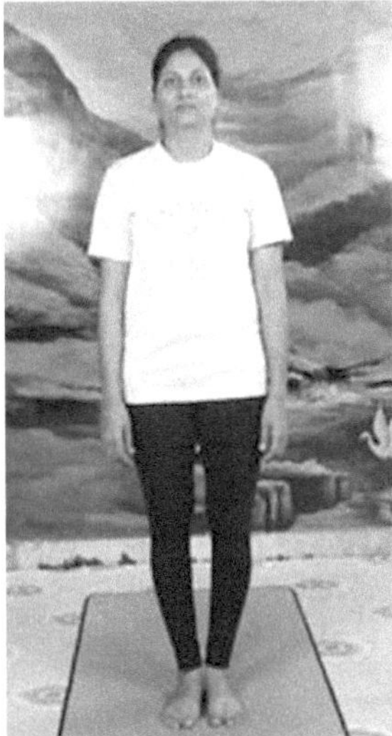

Step I

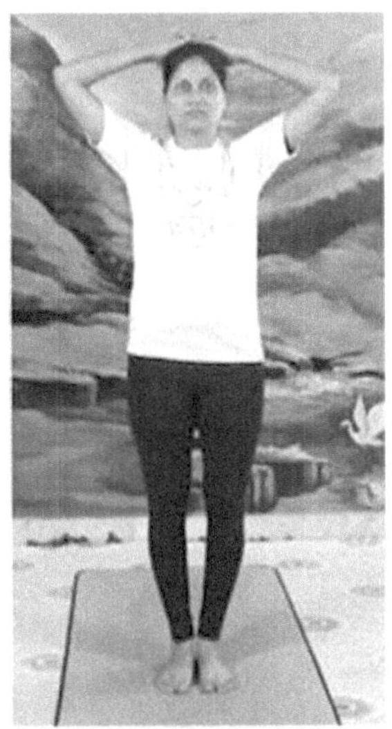

Step II

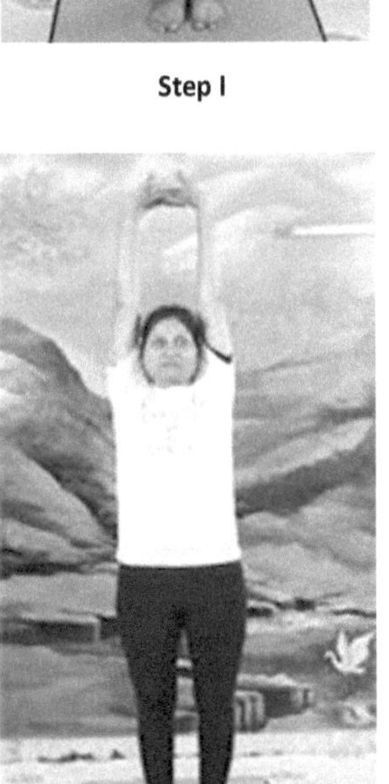

Final

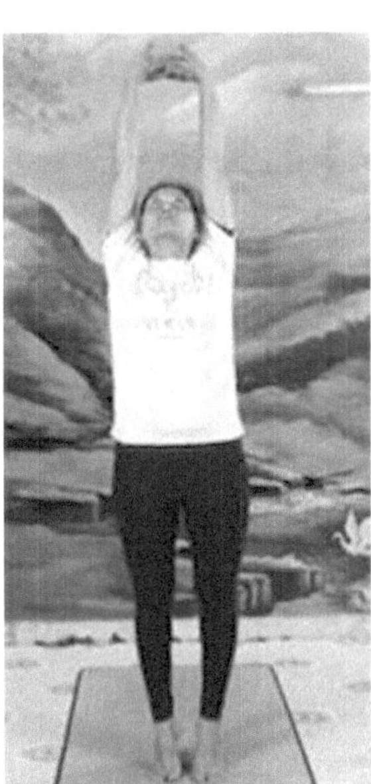

Advance

Stand erect, keeping the feet about half a foot or 15 cm apart. Interlock the fingers and place the hands on top of the head. Now turn your palm upward, raise and stretch your hand upward. Also, stretch the whole body upward rising up onto your tiptoes. After five seconds, lower your heels and arms to the starting position. Inhale while rising upward and exhale on returning. This is one round.

Triyak Tadasan
(Side Bending Palm Tree Pose)

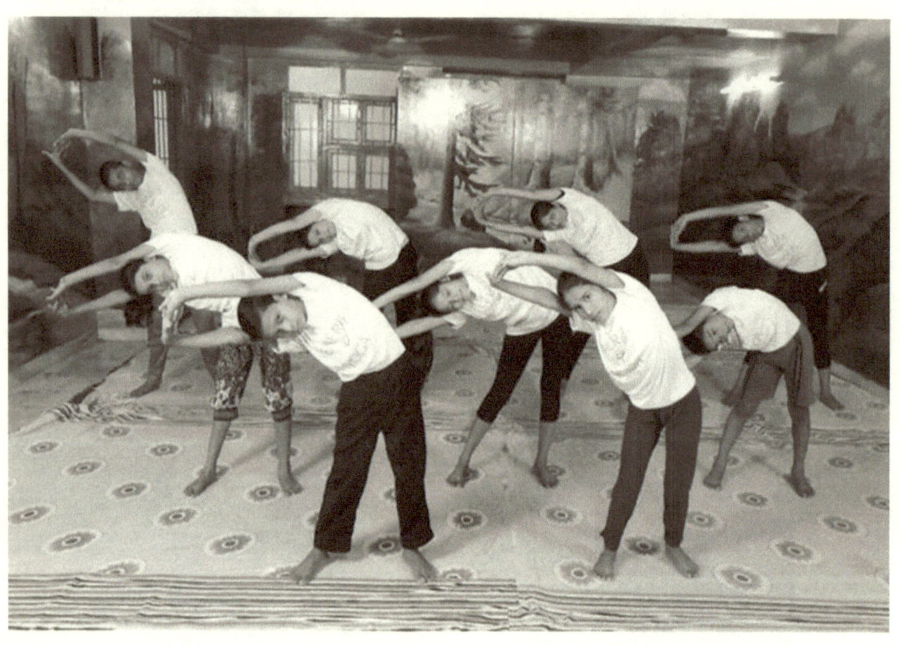

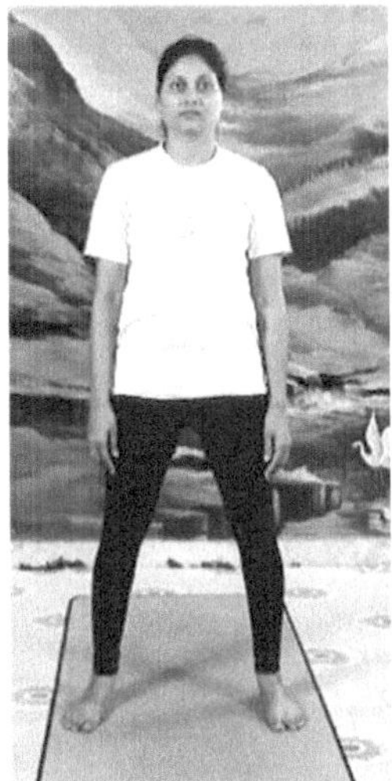

Step I

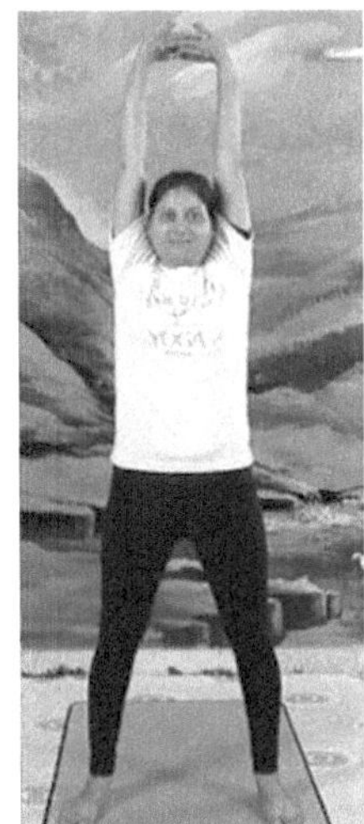

Step II

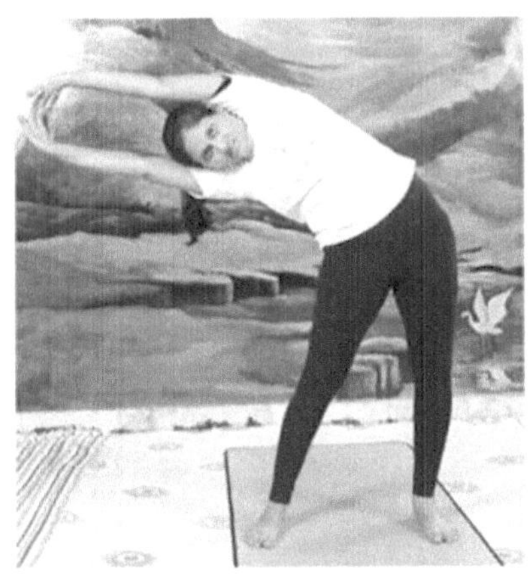

Step III

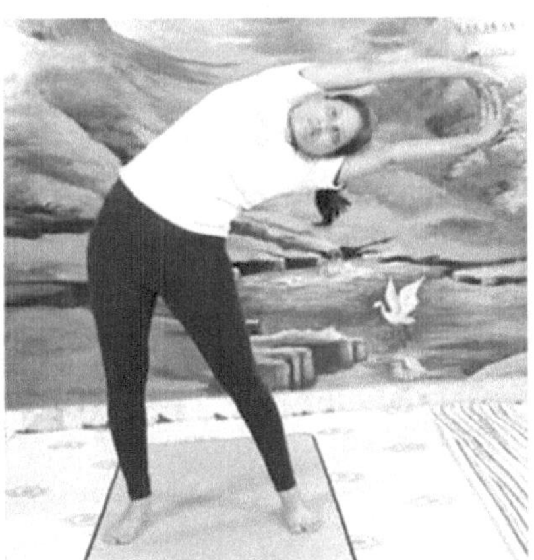

Step IV

For Triyak Tadasan, keep your feet 2 feet or 60 cm apart. Keeping hands and palms up bend the body towards right side. Hold 5 seconds, come in straight position and then bend the body towards the left and hold for 5 seconds. Exhale while bending and inhale while coming to the straight position. This is one round.

Kati Chakrasan
(Waist Rotating Pose)

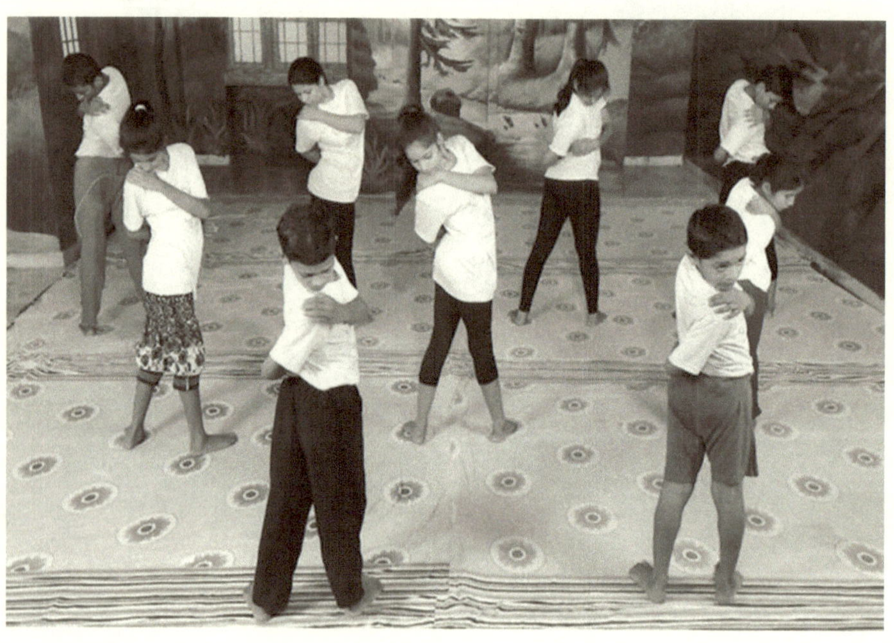

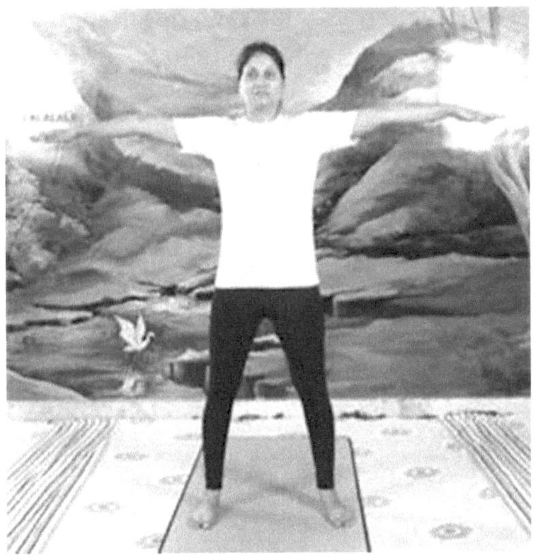

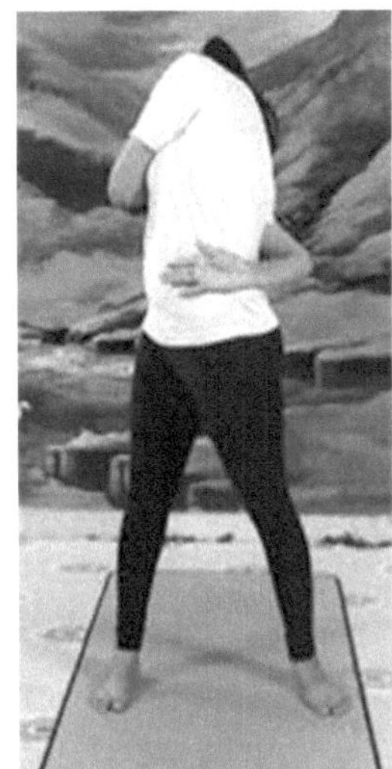

Step I

Step II

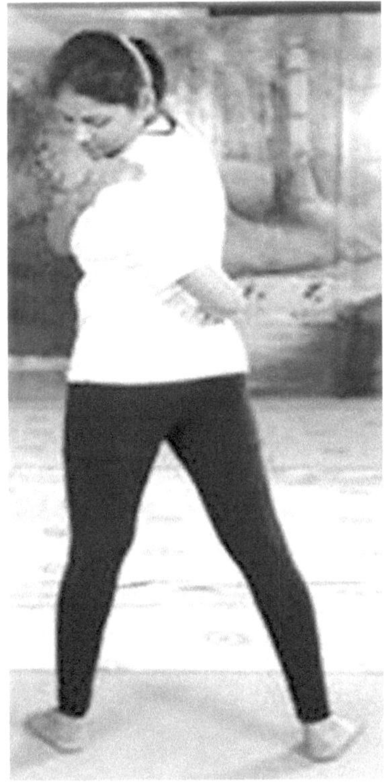

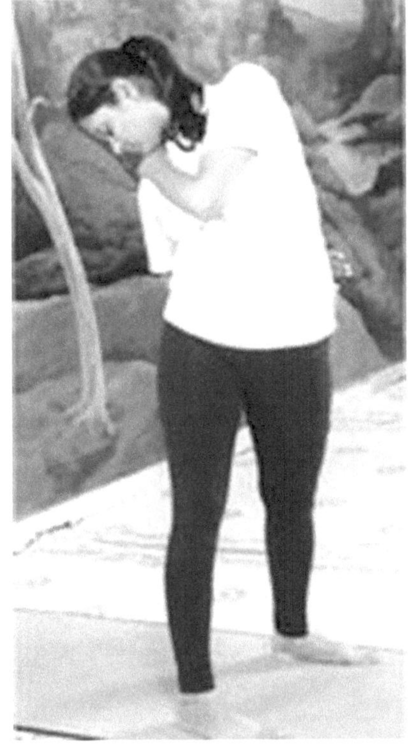

Step III

Step IV

With your feet about 2 feet or 60 cm apart, put your right hand on the left shoulder and left hand at the back, palm facing outwards. Exhale and Twist your upper part and abdomen to the left. Hold for 5 seconds. Inhale while returning and again exhale to repeat the same towards the right side. Again hold for 5 seconds. This is one round of Kati Chakrasan.

BENEFITS OF TTK

Tadasan, Triyak Tadasan and Kati Chakrasan are called TTK in short form. It releases tension of the spine and relaxes it. It is also good to increase the height of children.

Anulom-Vilom Pranayam
(Alternate Nostril Breathing)

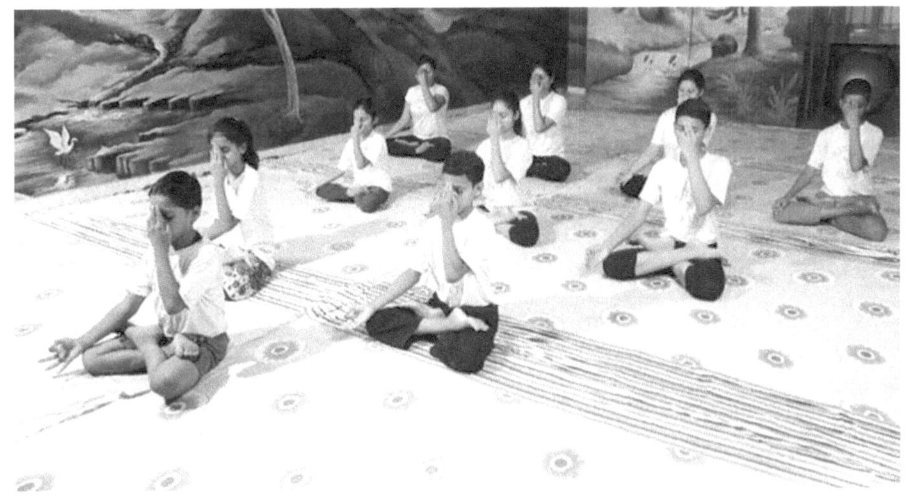

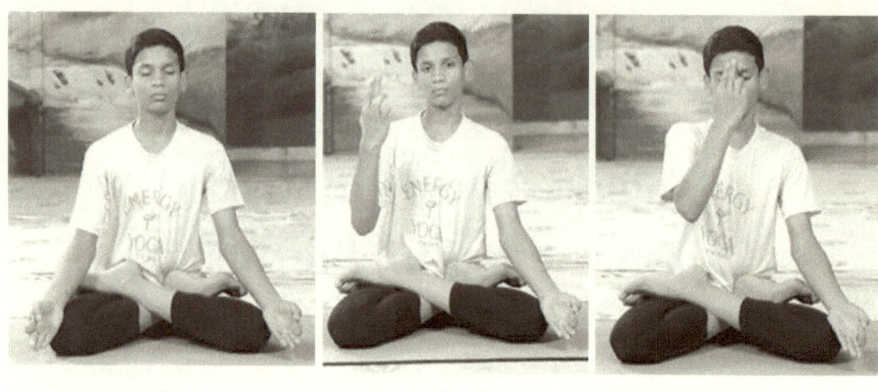

Step I   **Step II**   **Final**

Sit comfortably in any asana. Close your eyes and relax the whole body keeping the spine erect. Close your right nostril and inhale slowly and deeply with left nostril. Now close your left nostril and exhale slowly with right nostril. After exhaling, Inhale with the right nostril. Again, close your right nostril, exhale with left nostril.

OR

- **Inhale with Left nostril.**
- **Exhale with Right nostril.**
- **Inhale with Right nostril.**
- **Exhale with Left nostril.**

This is one round. Anulom-Vilom (Alternate) Pranayam is also called Nadi (Nerve) Shodhan (Purification) Pranayam. Thus it purifies the whole nervous system. Right nostril breathing stimulates the left hemisphere of the brain and left nostril breath activates the right hemisphere. Most diseases are caused by the imbalance between the two hemispheres of the brain. Left nostril is Ida, moon, cold, yin and right nostril is Pingala, Sun, Heat, and Yan. Through alternate breathing both hemispheres of the brain, as well as cold and heat get balanced.

Anulom-Vilom is the best Pranayam. It can be done even by bed ridden person, while lying on his bed. If you do not want to do different yogic activities, do only this Pranayam.

It has curative effects on all diseases, start with five rounds and prolong your practice up to sixty rounds according to your physical capacity.

Dhyan (Meditation)

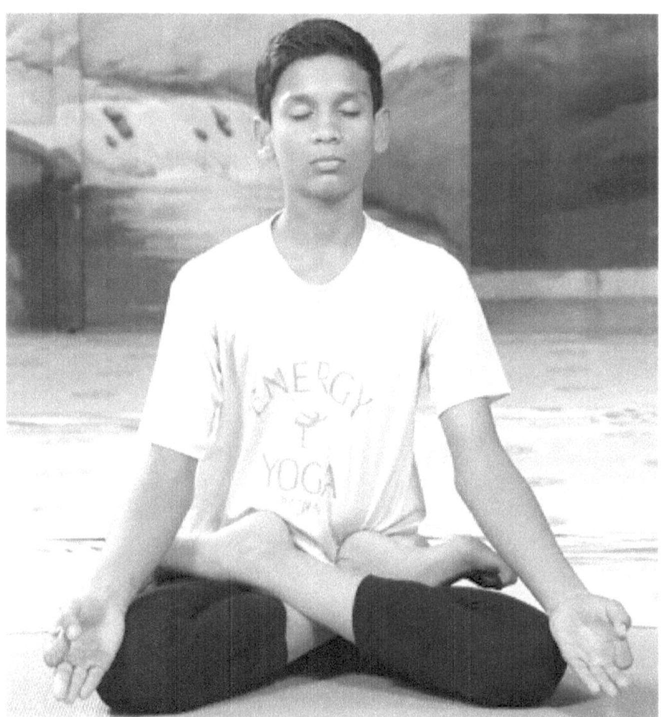

S it comfortably on any asana and close your eyes. Now visualize mentally that I am stilling my body and mind. With closed eyes see your whole body which is still and in peace. With closed eyes see your soles, ten fingers of legs, both legs, waist, whole back, spine , abdomen, navel, chest, both palms, all ten fingers, both hands, back and front of the neck, whole face, top of the head. Now see your whole body.

Bring your attention on your in and out breath and go on watching it like a gate keeper.

Meditation opens the flow of energy, relaxes you and keeps you healthy. It also saves you from natural calamities and destroys the bondages of karma (actions).

BEYOND ZERO MINUTE YOGA

Abdominal Breathing

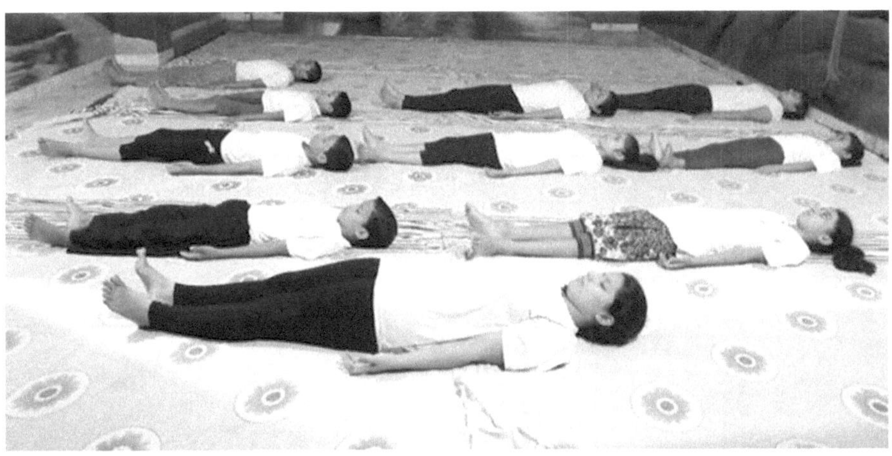

Lie in corpse pose (Shavasana). Shavasana itself is an important asana of relaxation. For corpse pose, lie flat on the back with the arms slightly apart from the body, half-open palms facing upward. Close your eyes and keep your feet slightly apart. Loosen your whole body and release its tension. Try to stop all your physical and mental movements. Remain in this state for some time and slowly come out of Shavasana.

Do Shavasana in between the asana practice, before you sleep or when you feel mentally or physically tired.

For abdominal breathing, lie in Shavasana and relax the whole body. Now inhale slowly while expanding the abdomen. Navel will go up while inhaling. Now exhale slowly and the abdomen will move downwards. Your chest and shoulders will remain still. Breathe slowly and deeply and feel the expansion and contraction of your abdomen.

Releasing physical tension is very important, because muscle tension can create disturbances in your body, affecting the whole system. Abdominal breathing is the natural way of breathing. It relaxes the whole system. It reduces the heart rate and lowers the blood pressure. In this world, which is full of stress and speed, abdominal breathing slows and calms the system. Corpse posture along with deep abdominal breathing increases longevity and fosters good health.

Agnisar Kriya

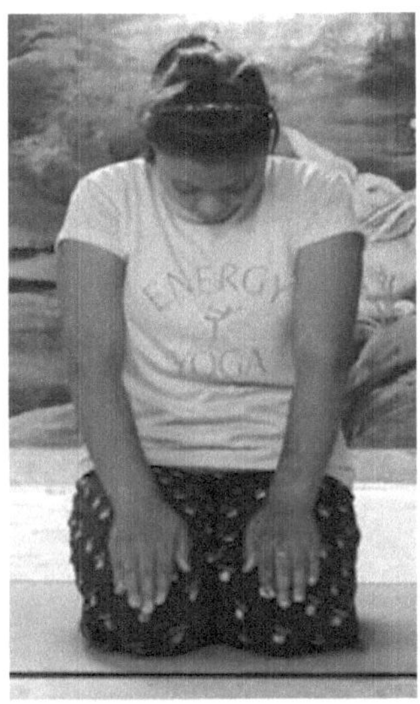

Sit in Vajrasana, Sukhasana or on a chair and place the palms of the hands on the knees. It can be done in standing position also by slightly bending the knees and the palms of the hands on the knees. Inhale, relax and finally exhale and bend your head forward so that the chin presses the neck. Now contract and release abdominal muscles rapidly for as long as it is possible to hold your breath outside comfortably. Straighten your head, relax it and take slow and deep breaths in. This is one round. Commence the next round. Do it for two to three rounds. Number of abdominal contractions per round will increase with the regular practice.

Agnisar Kriya massages and tones the entire abdominal area which includes the abdominal muscles, nerves, intestines, reproductive, urinary, and excretory organs. It stimulates the appetite and improves the digestion.

It is a powerful Kriya, so perform it cautiously and according to your physical capacity. It is not the part of ZMY, but looking at its benefit it has been given as an optional practice to do.

Nadis

The literal meaning of the word Nadi is 'flow' or 'current'. Sometimes it has been translated as 'nerve'. Nadis are the subtle channels through which the pranic forces flow. According to the yogic scriptures, there are 72000 nadis, or energy channels. Among them, Ida, Pingala, and Shushmna are the most important. Diseases are the manifestation of imbalance in nadis.

Ida opens in left nostril and known as Chandra or moon nadi. Pingala opens in right nostril and known as Surya or Sun nadi. Ida is cool, feminine, introvert and passive. Pingala, on the other hand, is heat, masculine, extrovert and active. During Ida phase or when the left nostril is flowing, the mind is introverted and suitable for undertaking mental work. During Pingala phase or when the right nostril is flowing, mind is extroverted and body generates more heat thus suitable for physical work and digestion. At the physical level, Ida corresponds to the parasympathetic nerve which relaxes the body and slows the heartbeat and respiration. Pingala corresponds to the sympathetic nerve which stimulates the body and accelerates the heartbeat and respiration.

The main purpose of yoga is to balance the flow of Ida and Pingala nadis. When Ida and Pingala nadis are purified, body becomes disease free and balanced which results in the flow of shushmna (central) nadi and thus opens the path of success in meditation.

Ayurveda

Ayurveda is the ancient Indian system of natural and holistic medicine. According to Ayurveda, each individual has prakriti or constitution. They are Kapha, Pitta and Vata. Every person is dominated by one constituent, and Ayurveda prescribes medicine or food according to the constitution of the body, whereas modern science gives emphasis on the nutrients of the food.

Though body has all the constituents and it remains healthy when all these constituents remain in their balance. Kapha (Cold) gives strength, Pitta (Heat) aids in digestion and makes active while Vata (air) circulates and manages the nutrients and waste products of the body. Imbalances in these constituents lead to illness.

Physical and mental traits of Kapha, Pitta and Vata dominated people are different from each other. Kapha dominated are overweight or heavy and easygoing, Pitta dominated are thin and irritable while Vata dominated are dry-skinned and nervous or fearful. Prakriti or constitution of the body remains constant for every individual for his or her lifetime. Disease tendency of an individual is decided by his or her Prakriti. Ayurvedic doctor decides medicine according to the Prakriti of the patient. The basic knowledge of Tridosha or Kapha, Pitta and Vata is also important for a Yogacharya (yoga teacher).

Panchakosha or Five Sheath

Yoga describes the body-mind complex of a man as consisting of five sheaths, or layers called Koshas. From gross to subtle they are Annamaya Kosha, Pranamaya Kosha, Manomaya Kosha, Vijnanamaya Kosha and Anandamaya Kosha.

Annamaya Kosha, foodstuff sheath, is the physical body and the first level of our experience. All physical activities like hunger and thirst, movement and interaction with the outer world are through Annamaya Kosha. The physical body or Annamaya Kosha has become the focal point of our attention and attraction in this world of consumerism.

Pranamaya Kosha, energy body, is the flowing energy or Prana or life force in the body. Eastern System gives much importance to the energy which is flowing in the body. Diseases occur due to energy blockage and when through different methods, the flow of energy is corrected the body becomes healthy and disease free. In the Chinese system, it is done through the manipulation of acupoints. All aspects of yoga – be it asana, pranayam or meditation corrects the energy circulation in the body.

Manomaya Kosha, mental body, is the layer of thought or mental experiences where likes, dislikes, needs, weaknesses, desires, ambitions etc., are processed. Awareness or mindfulness is the keyword in yoga which emphasises on being aware, on observing ourselves and to expand the field of Manomaya Kosha so that mental experiences can be perceived and stabilized in the right perspective.

Vijananamaya Kosha, intellect body, is the higher mental body which penetrates in the intuitive ability of the mind and remains conscious on the internal as well as the external level. The zone of Vijananamaya Kosha is reached when we transcend the boundary of rational and intellectual mind. There we find the unmanifested and subtle dimension of the mind and feel the intense self-awareness generated inside. These things happen in the state of deep meditation.

Anandamaya Kosha, bliss body, is the pure and radiant bliss body where conscious awareness is dropped and the fusion of the cosmic mind and the individual mind has taken place. The whole body becomes full of vitality, pleasure and happiness.

The purpose of yoga is to prepare the body and mind to access the deeper subtle Kosha layers. It is a journey from Annamaya Kosha to Anandamaya Kosha.

Shatkarma

Shatkarma means six practices of yogic purification. Before entering into the yogic practice, the body needs to be purified. Without purification, toxins accumulated in the body create many types of problems and illnesses after starting the advance yoga practice. Shatkarma removes the toxins and impurities of the body and mind and prepares it for further yogic practice. The Shatkarmas balance the three doshas or humours in the body: Kapha, mucus; Pitta, bile; and Vata, wind. The Shatkarmas are Neti, Dhauti, Nauli, Basti, Kapalbhati and Trataka.

Neti is nasal cleaning, the process of cleansing and purifying the nasal passage. It clears the sinuses which makes the area above the neck free and increases the optimum functioning of the optical and auditory nerves.

Dhauti is gentle washing with many forms, each having a specific purpose and reason. Through different types of dhauti, internal cleaning from the head to the anus is done. Important ones among them are:

- Varisara Dhauti (Shankha Prakshalan) to clean the intestines.
- Vahnisara Dhauti (Agnisar Kriya) activating the digestive fire.
- Vaman Dhauti (Kunjal)
  Cleaning the stomach by voluntary vomiting after drinking water. It removes excess acid or mucus.
- Vatsara Dhauti is the process of cleaning the stomach by swallowing the air through the mouth and expelling it through the anus after holding for some time. It helps to eliminate many stomach ailments.

Basti is a technique used for washing and toning the intestines and colon. It is close to modern process of enema. In Basti water or air is sucked into the anus using some yogic techniques. The water or air is retained inside for some time and then allowing it to flow back out again.

Nauli is the rotation of stomach muscles. Nauli has a very powerful effect on the physical body. Nauli is an advance practice which can be done only after doing some preparatory practices like Agnisar and Uddiyan Bandha.

Kapalbhati is frontal brain cleansing. Mental burdens are cleared through Kapalbhati. Three popular methods are Vatkarma Kapalbhati (air cleansing), Vyutkrama Kapalbhati (Sinus Cleansing) and Sheetkarma Kapalbhati (mucus cleansing)

Trataka is intense gazing at one point or object. It develops the optimum concentration and awareness.

Thus Shatkarmas clean and activate the body at physical, pranic and mental level and prepare it for higher level of yogic practices.

Eight Stages of Patanjali

Patanjali's yoga sutra for the first time codified the comprehensive system of yoga often called as the eight fold path of yoga, a non-sectarian yoga. They are Yama, Niyama, Asana, Pranayam, Pratyahara, Dharana, Dhyan and Samadhi. The first four stages are the external aspects through which the external stimulation and the environment are controlled. Through the last four stages, mind is withdrawn and the further inputs of impressions are stopped into the field of consciousness.

Yama (social code) is comprised of ahinsa (non-violence), satya (Truthfulness), asteya (honesty), aparigraha (non-acquisitiveness) and brahmacharya (celibacy but actually it means 'one who is established in higher consciousness').

Niyama (Personal code) comprises sauch (cleanliness), santosha (contentment) tapas (austerity), swadhaya (self-study) and ishwara pranidhana (cultivation of faith).

These five yamas and five niyamas eliminate the problems of the mind. The negative influences on the emotional, psychic and mental bodies embedded in the deepest recesses of the consciousness are removed.

Asana is a physical posture, in which one is at total ease and steady.

Pranayam is the regulation of breath.

Asana and Pranayam are not discussed in detail by Patanjali.

Pratyahara is withdrawing the mind from external stimuli. It is the first stage of internalising the mind.

Dharana means to hold or bind the mind at one point. The word used in Yoga sutra is 'Samapatti' or absorption.

Dhyana-Prolonged period of dharana leads to the next stage called Dhyana, when the mind succeeds in keeping itself in that state for some time.

Samadhi – When that, giving up all forms, reflects only the meaning, it is Samadhi. When the aim of meditation is realized without involvement of personal consciousness, it is known as the state of Samadhi.

Chakra

Yoga emphasises on the subtle aspects of the body and the flow of energy in the body. The chakras are the vortices of pranic energy at specific areas in the body. There are seven important chakras located along the pathway of Sushumna, an energy channel which flows through the centre of the spinal cord. On a physical level, chakras are closely associated with the major nerve plexuses and endocrine glands in the body. The purpose of yoga is to move the energy upward from the lowest chakra to the highest chakra or from the gross to the subtle.

Muladhar chakra is the root chakra and is situated at the perineum in the male body and at the cervix in the female body. It is the seat or dwelling place of primal energy or Kundalini Shakti represented as a red serpent coiled three and a half times around the linga. Through different yogic methods serpent is activated to move upward.

Swadhisthana Chakra or 'one's own abode' is situated two fingers width above the Muladhar chakra. It is the seat of most primitive and deep rooted instincts.

Manipura Chakra or 'city of jewels' is situated in the spine behind the navel and chiefly concerned with the vital process of digestion and food metabolism.

Anahata Chakra or 'unstuck' is situated in the spine, behind the sternum, level with the heart. It is associated with emotions and unconditional love.

Vishuddhi Chakra or 'Purification' is situated at the back of the neck, behind the throat pit. It is a place where physical, psychic and mental purification occurs.

Ajna Chakra or 'command' is situated in the midbrain, behind the place between the eyebrows (bhrumadhya) at the top of the spine. It is associated with wisdom and intuition.

Sahasrara Chakra or 'one thousand' is situated at the crown of head. It is here, where everything merges into pure consciousness.

These chakras are very powerful energy centres and each chakra represents a certain behaviour, thought or emotional pattern. A yoga therapist can advise his patient to meditate on certain chakras to cure diseases.

Nada

The word Nada means flow, but generally it means sound. According to the Nada Yoga, the universe is the projection of sound vibrations. The Upanishads and the Vedas describe that in the beginning was nothing, there was only sound. From that sound, the universe evolved, and therefore the fundamental structure of the universe is based on nada or sound vibrations.

Adi Sankaracharya in Yoga Taravali regards nada as the highest form of meditation. He says 'O contemplation on Nada! Salutations to you. I know you to be the means to attain the truth. By your grace, my mind, together with breath, dissolves in the supreme state.'

"In the beginning was the word, and the word was with God and the word was God." (New Testament, the Gospel of St John).

Patanjali in yogasutra also emphasises the importance of Pranava or sacred sound as the manifestation of the universe.

The Sufis or Muslim mystics called it Sruti, in Sikhism it is shabda. Kabirdas, Gorakhnath and many other mystics regarded the sound or vibration as the source of the universe. References of sound are found in many ancient religions and cultures.

The Kashmir Saiva school holds that the ultimate reality itself 'quivers' that is inherently creative. The absolute is a throb (Spanda) which vibrates as the primordial sound (nada). "Spanda is the pulsation of the ecstasy of the divine consciousness" as Abhinava Gupta defines it. When we sense this pulsation inside us, we are sensing our own personal spark of that huge, primordial life force.

The superstring theory emphasises the vibratory nature of creation. According to string theory, there is only one fundamental ingredient – the string. Each arises from a different vibrational pattern executed by the same underlying entity. Dr Michio Kaku says that God could be a mathematician:

"The mind of God we believe is cosmic music, the music of strings resonating through eleven dimensional hyperspace. That is the mind of God."

There are four stages of manifestation of sound from the subtle to the gross level. These four stages are Para, Pashyanti, Madhyama and Vaikhari.

Para nada means 'transcendental', 'beyond' or 'the other side'. It is Kundalini Sakti (Power). It is the central creative power of the entire sound of all the subjective and objective phenomena. It is beyond the reach of the indriyas, or sense organs.

Pashyanti means 'that which can be seen or visualised'. The ancient scriptures maintain that sound can be perceived. Pashyanti is that where the word and the object are identical. The division between word and object has not yet arisen. It consists of one anu (Part). It is said to be existing in the heart.

Madhyama means 'in between' or 'middle', so madhyama means a middle sound. In the madhyama stage, though the division between the word and object has started, it is not fully pronounced yet. It is of two anus (parts) and resides in the throat.

Vaikhari or Vikhara means body. The body is the seat of gross speech and therefore it is known as vaikhari. In the vaikhari stage the object is completely separated from the word. It is said to exist in the root of the tongue and consists of three anus (Parts).

The aim of meditation on nada or sound is to find out the primal, the finest the ultimate sound. The process starts from the external gross sound, and the transcendental form of sound is conceivable only through going into the deeper realms of our consciousness.

Some Advance Asanas

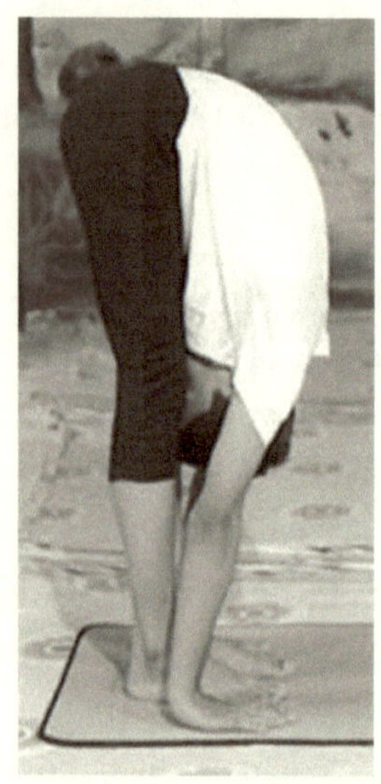
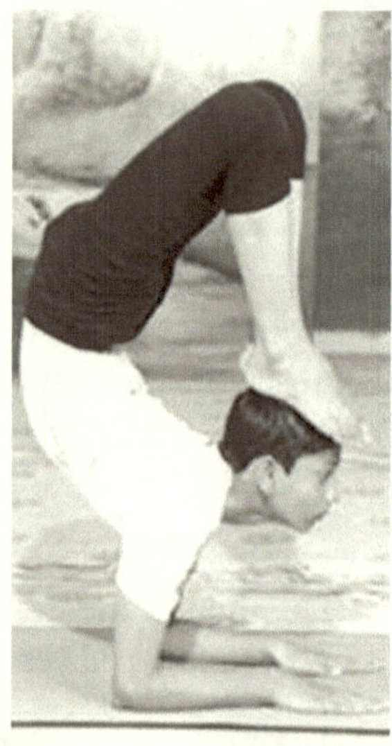
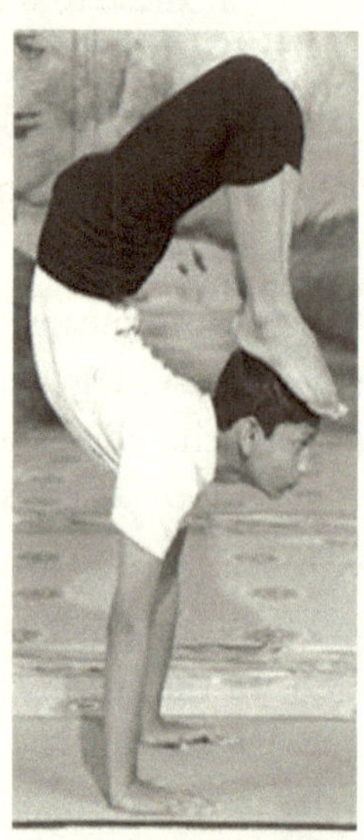
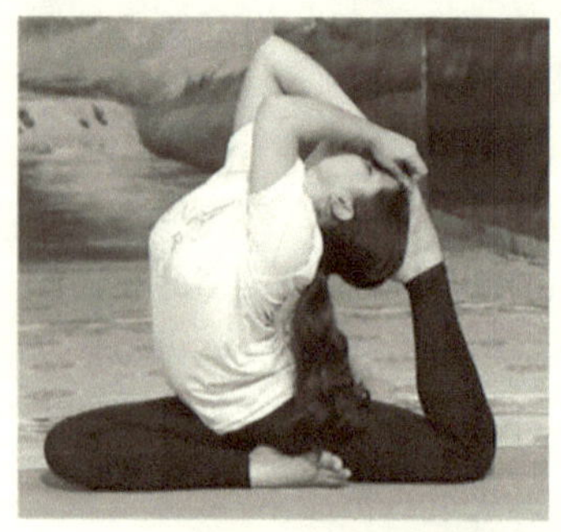
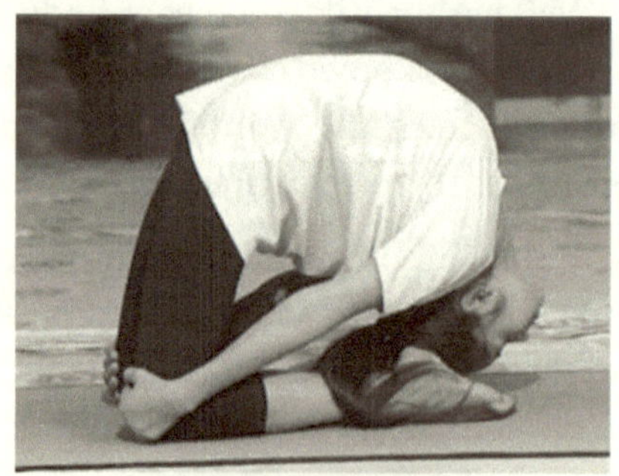
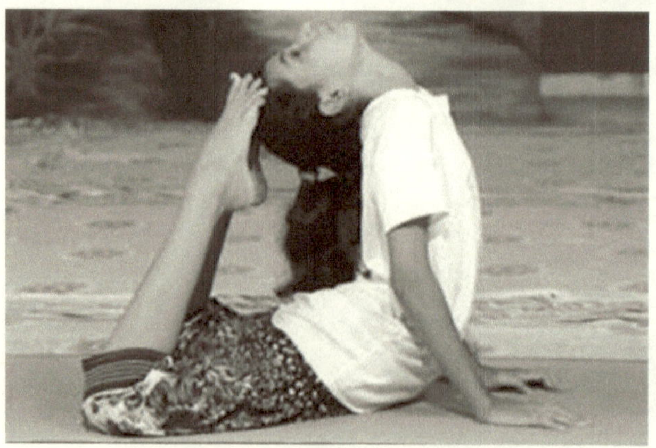

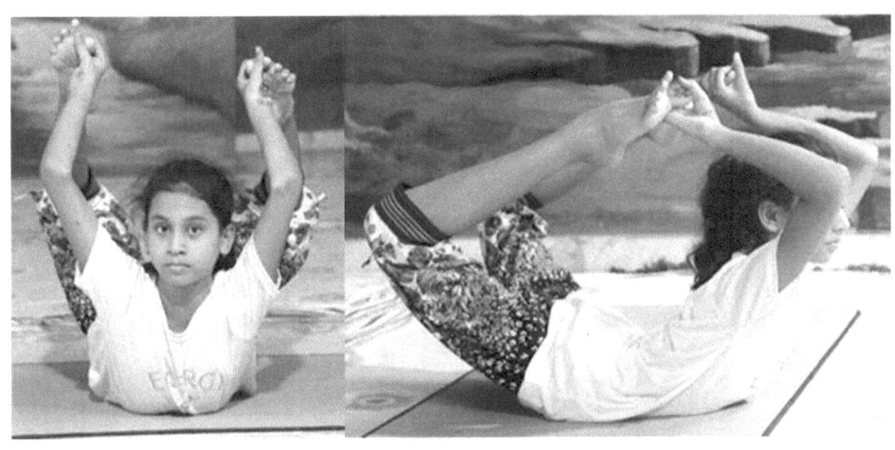

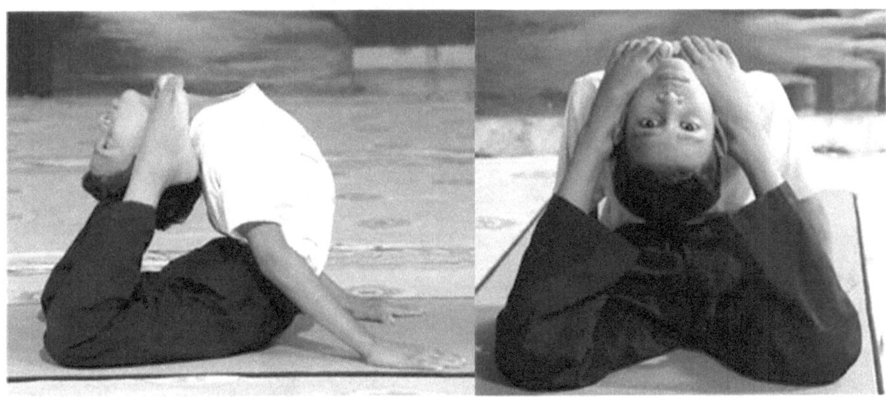

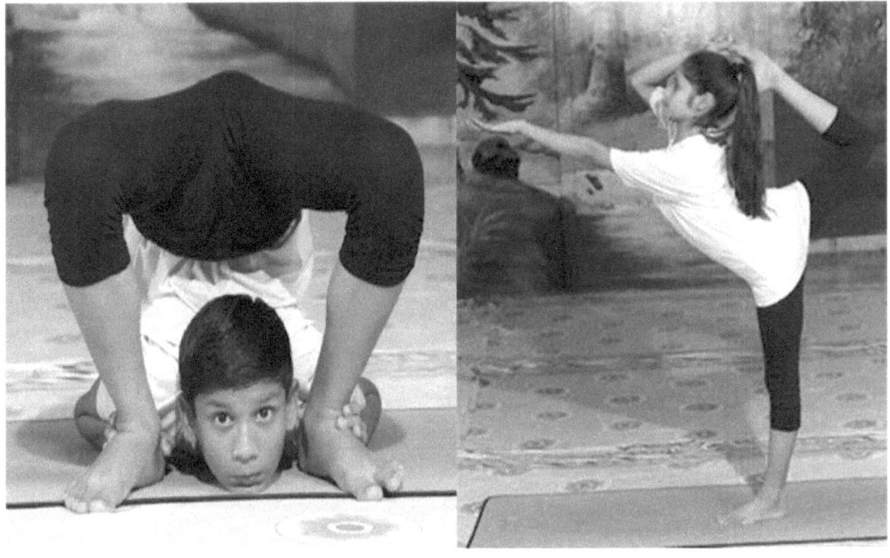

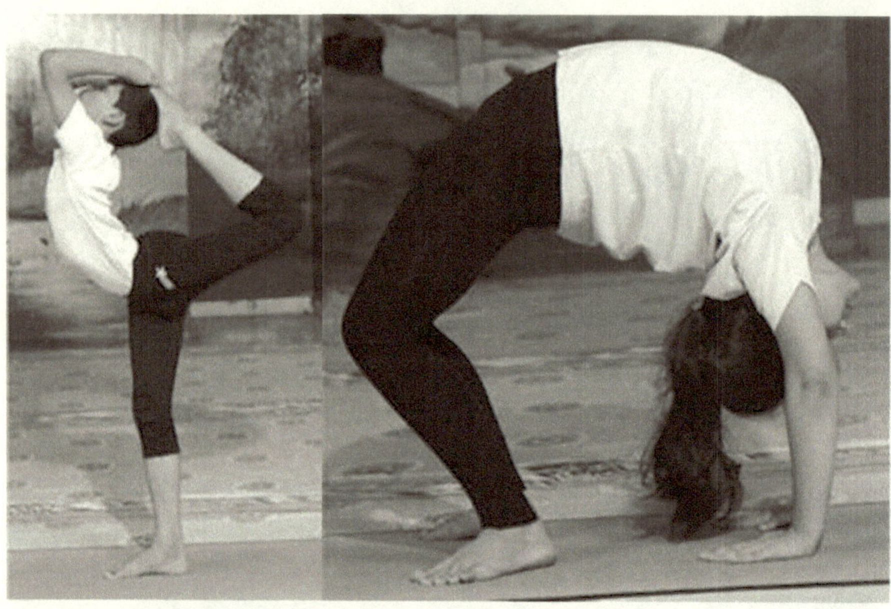

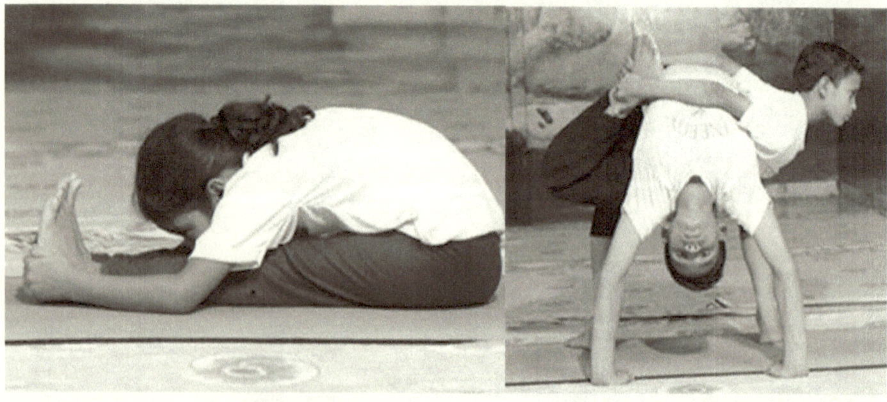

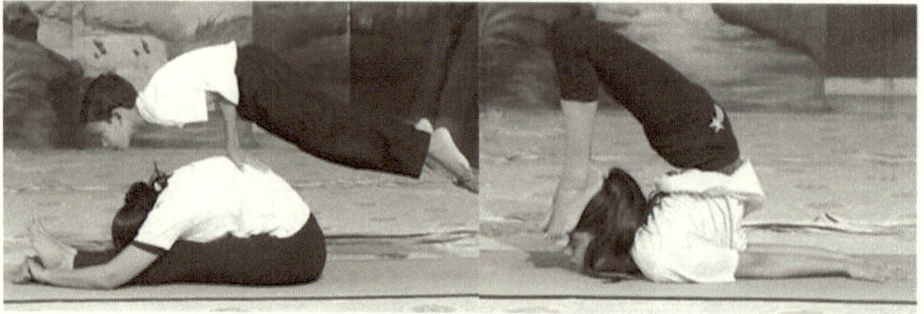

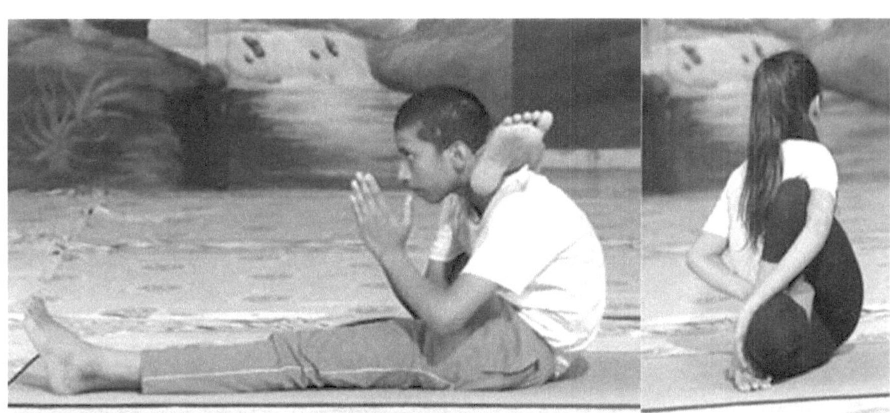

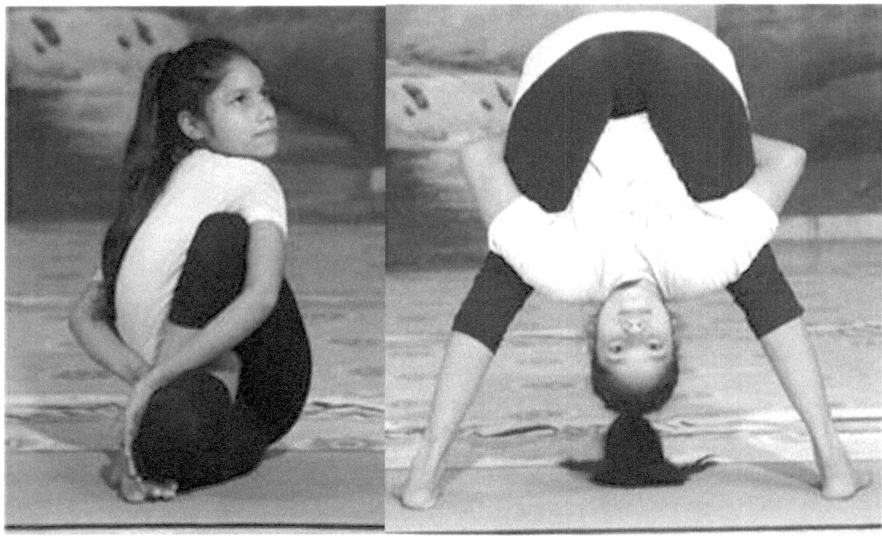

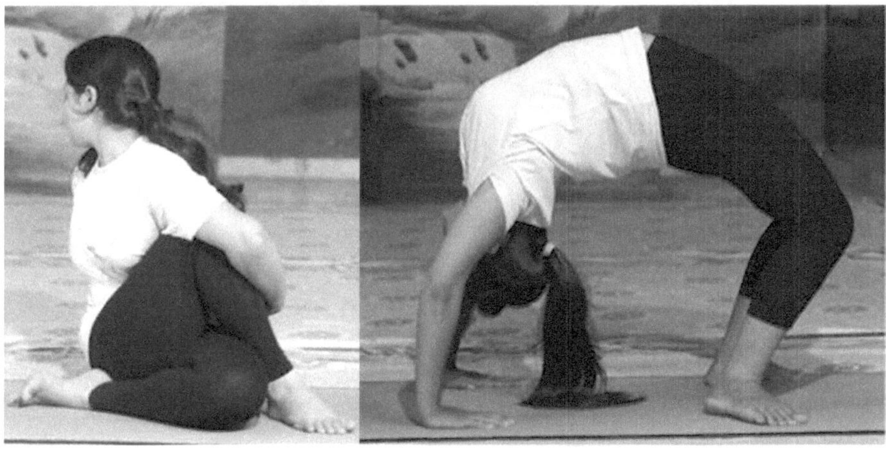

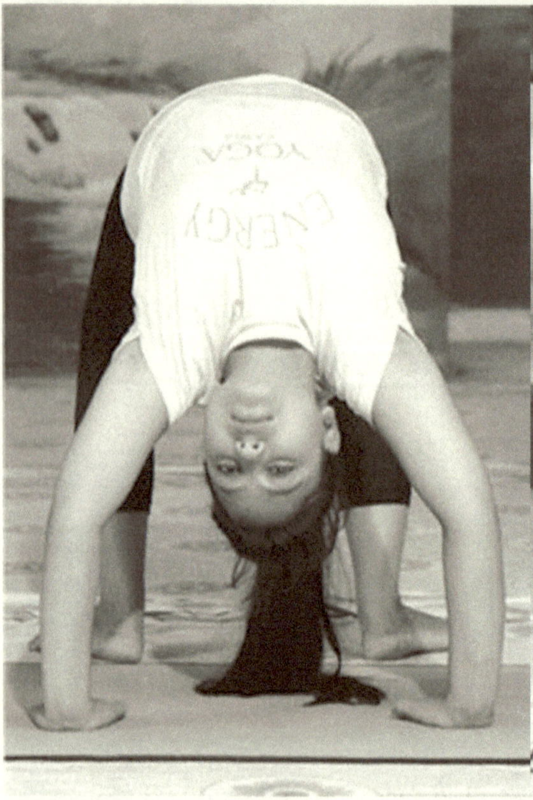

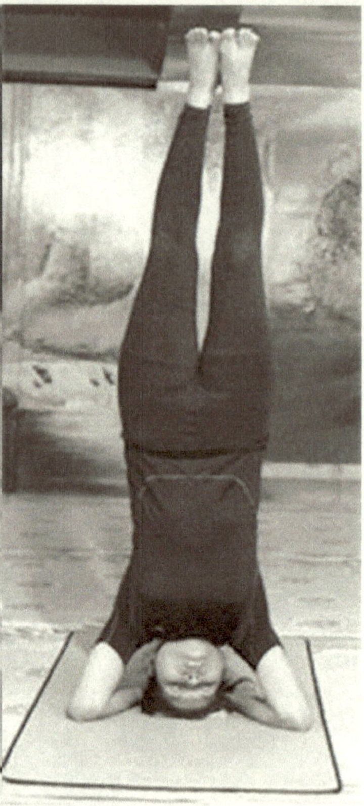

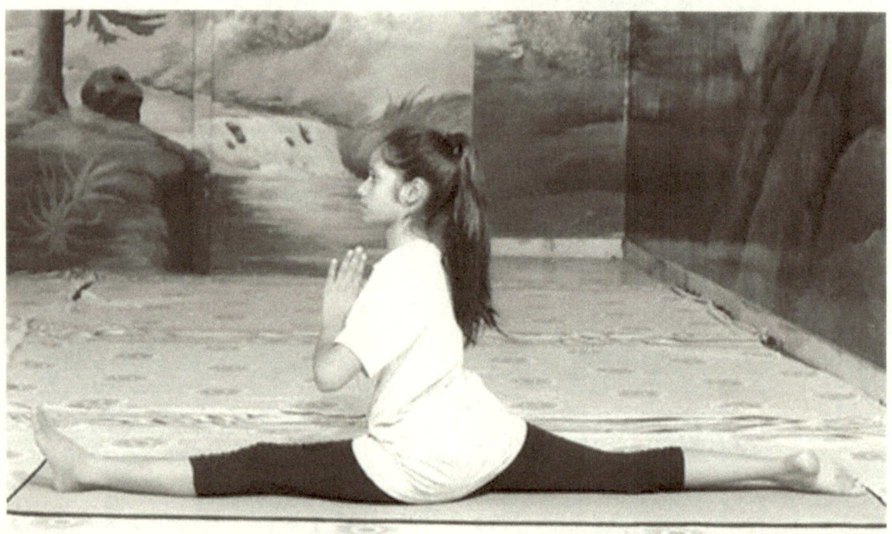

"Aamkumbh Ivamvastho Jiryamanh Sada Ghatah
Yogalen Sandhay Ghat Sudh in Sadacharetah"

—Gheranda Sanhita

The body wears away like a raw earthen jar,
Make it strong by baking it in the fire of yoga.

www.ingramcontent.com/pod-product-compliance
Lightning Source LLC
Chambersburg PA
CBHW051414250726
48655CB00003B/1036